Flaxseed and Flaxseed Oil
3rd Edition

Kate Gilbert Udall

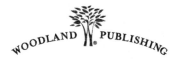

WOODLAND PUBLISHING

For permissions, ordering information, or bulk quantity discounts, contact:
Woodland Publishing, Salt Lake City, Utah
Visit our website: www.woodlandpublishing.com
Toll-free number: (800) 777-BOOK

The information in this book is for educational purposes only and is not recommended as a means of diagnosing or treating an illness. All matters concerning physical and mental health should be supervised by a healthcare practitioner knowledgeable in treating that particular condition. Neither the publishers nor the author directly or indirectly dispenses medical advice, nor do they prescribe any remedies or assume any responsibility for those who choose to treat themselves.

Cataloging-in-Publication data is available from the Library of Congress

ISBN: 978-1-58054-203-6

Printed in the United States of America

Contents

Ancient Seed   5

Essential Fatty Acids (EFAs)   6

    Functions of EFAs   6

    Omega-3 and Omega-6   7

    Negative Effects of a Fatty Acid Imbalance   9

Flaxseed: Triple the Benefits   10

Fish Oil vs. Flaxseed and Flaxseed Oil   10

Flaxseed and Lignans   11

Flaxseed and Fiber   12

Health Benefits of Flaxseed   13

    Heart Disease   13

    High Cholesterol   14

    High Blood Pressure   16

    Stroke   16

    Rheumatoid Arthritis   17

    Multiple Sclerosis   18

    Psoriasis   18

    Cancer   19

    Attention Deficit Hyperactivity Disorder   20

    Additional Roles of Flaxseed and Flaxseed Oil   21

Continuing Research   23

Selecting a Flaxseed Source   24

    Choosing a Good Flaxseed Oil   24

    Tips for Storing and Using Whole or Ground Flaxseed   25

Precautions with Whole and Ground Flaxseed   26

Dosing   26

Promote Whole Body Health   27

References   28

Ancient Seed

Since ancient times, people have harvested and used flaxseed and flaxseed oil in their diets. Flax, a blue flowering plant with oil-rich seeds, originated in Egypt in about 5000 BC. Flax was extremely important to ancient Egyptians, who used flax fibers to spin linen for clothing in addition to consuming flaxseed and flaxseed oil for nutritional and medicinal (primarily laxative) purposes. Flax fibers come from the plant's stalk; edible flaxseeds are the "fruit" of the flax plant. Flax plants produce several small, round capsules that contain flaxseeds. When pressed, flaxseeds produce flaxseed oil, also called linseed oil.

Cultures other than the Egyptians recognized flaxseed and flaxseed oil for their medicinal value. In 650 BC, ancient Greek physician Hippocrates wrote about using flaxseed to relieve abdominal pain. In the eighth century AD, Roman Emperor Charlemagne considered flaxseed so important to health that he passed laws requiring his subjects to consume it. Rations for Charlemagne's army included flaxseed.

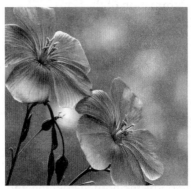

Flax is a blue flowering crop, grown since ancient times for its health benefits.

Even though early peoples may not have known what natural properties of flaxseed made it such a valuable part of their diet, they recognized that flaxseed and flaxseed oil possessed healthful qualities. Modern research backs ancient wisdom about the value of flaxseed. Although research about flaxseed is ongoing, many recent studies suggest exciting health benefits of both flaxseed and flaxseed oil. Flaxseed shows promise in helping to prevent and manage heart disease, cancer, rheumatoid arthritis, multiple sclerosis, attention deficit hyperactivity disorder (ADHD) and more!

Essential Fatty Acids (EFAs)

In order to understand why flaxseed and flaxseed oil are beneficial, it is important to understand a little about *essential fatty acids*, or EFAs. Fats are composed of a variety of fatty acids, which are an important energy source for cells in the body. Not all fatty acids are "essential," however. A fatty acid is considered "essential" if it is necessary for health, but the body cannot produce it.

Only two types of fatty acids are considered essential to the human diet—alpha-linolenic acid and linoleic acid. Both EFAs come from plant sources. The body can produce other fatty acids, such as EPA and DHA (which will be discussed later) from the two essential fatty acids, meaning that EPA and DHA are not considered "essential," even though they are also important to good health.

When the body does not have a sufficient supply of fatty acids, deficiency symptoms can develop. Symptoms of a fatty acid deficiency include:

- dry hair and hair loss
- dry skin
- slow wound healing
- impaired ability to learn and recall information
- dermatitis (itchy, painful inflammation of the skin)
- increased susceptibility to infection
- stiff/painful joints

Functions of EFAs

Fatty acids are important to the body for three main reasons. First, body tissues use EFAs to produce *prostaglandins*, important fat compounds that are similar to hormones. Prostaglandins are produced throughout the entire body and function as messenger molecules, transmitting information to mediate cell responses. Prostaglandins perform a variety of functions in the body, including widening and narrowing blood vessels, secreting gastric acid, regulating hormones and calcium and mediating inflammation. A fatty acid deficiency can disrupt the body's balance of prostaglandins, setting into motion undesirable (and often harmful) physical effects.

The second reason EFAs are essential is that they are vital to the membrane structure of all the body's cells. Essential fatty acids are incorporated into a fatty layer of cell membranes called the *phospholipid bilayer*. As part of the phospholipid bilayer, EFAs help keep cell membranes flexible and permeable so that nutrients can flow into cells and waste materials can flow out.

The third reason EFAs are essential involves the activities of *enzymes* bound in the cell membranes. Enzymes are catalysts that activate chemical reactions throughout the body. Life would not exist without enzymes. The body is made of trillions of cells, all of which require enzymes to function. Having an adequate amount of EFAs to support cell properties and functions is essential for energy production, cell repair and detoxification, all functions initiated by enzymes.

Omega-3 and Omega-6

Fatty acids are categorized as omega-3s or omega-6s. A fatty acid is placed in one of the categories according to its chemical structure. Omega-3s and omega-6s come from different sources and perform different functions in the body. In general, omega-6s tend to increase inflammation, which is an essential part of the body's immune response. However, chronic (prolonged) inflammation can damage healthy blood vessels and joints, causing disease. Omega-3s help prevent complications associated with inflammation by decreasing inflammation. Both omega-6 and omega-3 fatty acids are necessary for optimum health.

The nutritionally important omega-3s include alpha-linolenic acid, found in plant seed oils, and ecosapentaenoic acid (EPA) and docosahexaenoic acid (DHA), found in fish, krill, calamari and algal oils. Alpha-linolenic acid is the *essential* fatty acid of the three because the body cannot produce it. Alpha-linolenic acid is the precursor to EPA and DHA, which means the body can produce EPA and DHA from dietary sources of alpha-linolenic acid. Even though EPA and DHA play a vital role in the development of the brain and eyes and are needed for cardiovascular health, they are not considered "essential" because the body is able to synthesize them from alpha-linolenic acid.

Recent research has also established that EPA and DHA, the fatty acids produced from alpha-linolenic acid, have anti-inflammatory properties and synthesize certain anti-inflammatory prostaglandins that offer protective effects against both coronary heart disease and stroke. Such fatty acids may be helpful in improving cardiovascular function, including lowering cholesterol levels and blood pressure. Omega-3 fatty acids may also benefit individuals who suffer from migraines and arthritis. And an analysis published in *Cancer* in 2011 suggests that EPA from fish oil helps prevent muscle wasting and weight loss in cancer patients undergoing chemotherapy.

Whether consumed from fish oil or as alpha-linolenic acid from flaxseed, omega-3s are necessary for the health of multiple body systems. In general, however, most Americans do not eat enough cold-water fish to adequately provide the necessary amount of EPA-DHA omega-3 fatty acids, nor do they consume adequate amounts of seeds high in alpha-linolenic acid to provide adequate amounts of omega-3 fatty acids. Flaxseed can help fill the void.

The other *essential* fatty acid, linoleic acid, is in the omega-6 category. Linoleic acid is derived from the Greek word *linon* for flax and is also found in flaxseed and flaxseed oil. It is an unsaturated fatty acid that the body can convert to arachidonic acid (AA), another omega-6 fatty acid found in cell membranes. Arachidonic acid is involved in growth of muscle tissue and in cell signaling, which is important to cell function. Arachidonic acid is also involved in early brain development and is a key building block for prostaglandins, which help destroy invading microorganisms. Such functions make both linolenic acid and AA omega-6 fatty acids beneficial in the treatment of certain skin conditions and a likely tool in successful growth and development therapies.

The human body relies on adequate dietary supplies of linoleic and alpha-linolenic acids to help all the cells in the body function normally. Flaxseed and flaxseed oil contain more than 50 percent alpha-linolenic acid and about 24 percent linoleic acid. Supplementing the diet with flaxseed and flaxseed oil is a great source of both linoleic and alpha-linolenic acids.

Flaxseed oil is extremely sensitive to light, heat and oxygen. Left at room temperature, the oil contained in flaxseed oil or ground flaxseed can quickly oxidize and turn rancid. Whole flaxseed is safe to store at room temperature as its thick shell insulates the oil inside from environmental oxygen, but ground flaxseed or flaxseed oil must be refrigerated.

Negative Effects of a Fatty Acid Imbalance

The standard American diet is deficient in omega-3 fatty acids. Nutrition experts recommend consuming four times more omega-6 fatty acids than omega-3s, a ratio of 4:1. However, the ratio in the diet of most Americans is 20:1 (and often, even higher)—meaning that most people consume 20 times more omega-6 fatty acids than omega-3 fatty acids (about five times the recommended amount).

Such an imbalance has numerous negative effects. An imbalance in omega-6 and omega-3 fatty acid intake increases the potential for chronic inflammation that is connected to diseases such as atherosclerosis (thickening of the artery walls), thrombosis (blood clot formation) and other vascular conditions, arthritis, asthma and some cancerous tumors. Maintaining a better ratio by increasing intake of omega-3 fatty acids can noticeably improve the function of the body.

Dr. William E. Connor, a scientist and clinician known for his research on the link between diet and disease as well as work on the benefits of omega-3s, noted, "It is probable . . . that there has always been the proper balance between these two groups of essential fatty acids, but in the modern era with the provision of inexpensive vegetable oils, it is possible that the pendulum for increased dietary omega-6 fatty acids in the form of linoleic acid has swung too far and the intake of omega-3 acids has actually declined."

An omega-3 imbalance with omega-6 produces a competitive interaction that can affect omega-3 conversions. Depending on the severity, such an imbalance can produce minor deficiencies or major disease states. Minor signs of omega-3 deficiency include skin dryness, goose flesh on the backs of the arms, loss of hair and changes in immune function, such as an increased susceptibility to infection. More serious imbalances caused by the overconsumption of omega-6 fatty acids can result in chronic inflammation, hypertension and blood clots, all of which elevate the risk for heart attack and stroke.

Because omega-6 fatty acids are usually found more abundantly in American diets, many people need to focus on finding better sources of omega-3 fatty acids. A unique feature of flaxseed is its high ratio of alpha-linolenic acid (omega-3) to linoleic acid (omega-6). Flaxseed and flaxseed oil have a ratio of about 4:1 of omega-6 fatty acids to omega-3 fatty acids, exactly in line with the optimum ratio recommended by nutritionists.

In response to research indicating flaxseed's potential health benefits, consumer demand for flaxseed and flaxseed oil is steadily increasing. Food manufacturers add ground flaxseed to foods ranging from frozen waffles to breads, pastas, oatmeal and more. Agricultural demand has also increased, as some farmers feed flaxseed to chickens so the chickens will produce healthier eggs. Chickens and other animals that are primarily fed grain tend to have high omega-6 concentrations, which they pass along to the humans that consume them. Adding flaxseed to a chicken's diet increases the chicken's omega-3 concentrations, which the chickens also pass along to humans.

Flaxseed: Triple the Benefits

Flaxseed is one of the few plant sources that contain essential omega-3 fatty acids in significant amounts. Flaxseed also has benefits that flaxseed oil does not have. Flaxseed's incredible potential comes from three components: omega-3 fatty acids, lignans and fiber. *Lignans* are phytoestrogens that may help prevent or manage breast cancer, prostate cancer and colon cancer. Some manufacturers process flaxseed oil so it retains particles of the seed coat, which contains the phytoestrogenic lignans. However, flaxseed oil does not normally contain lignans unless the label specifies that it does. (Learn more about the benefits of lignans on page 11.)

In addition to lignans, flaxseed (but not flaxseed oil) is an excellent source of dietary fiber, which is a vital component in a healthy diet. Because of its high fiber content, flaxseed is an excellent remedy for constipation. (Learn more about the benefits of dietary fiber in flaxseed on page 12.)

Fish Oil vs. Flaxseed and Flaxseed Oil

Studies suggest that flaxseed and flaxseed oil, like fish oil, offer many benefits in fighting disease and improving overall health. But should you choose fish oil or flaxseed oil? First of all, remember that flaxseed contains a different type of omega-3 fatty acids than fish oil. Flaxseed and flaxseed oil contain alpha-linolenic acid, while fish oils are composed of EPA and DHA. The body can use alpha-linolenic acid to manufacture EPA and DHA. In other words, the body converts the oils in flaxseed oils into the same fatty acids found in fish oil.

While some people prefer to take fish oil to get EPA and DHA directly, people who are vegetarian, vegan or allergic to fish cannot take fish oil. For such individuals, flaxseed oil and flaxseed are an excellent way to get the omega-3 fatty acids that the body needs. Other advantages include:

- Taste and smell is more pleasant—no more "fish burps"!
- Flaxseed is a three-in-one: a good source of fiber, omega-3s *and* lignans.
- Lignans may be beneficial for women needing more phytoestrogens at menopause.
- Flaxseed oil can be added to smoothies, yogurt or other foods or beverages while fish oil softgels can't be added!

Flaxseed and Lignans

While the fatty acids found in flaxseed and flaxseed oil are important to health, the lignans found in flaxseed also demonstrate impressive health benefits. Lignans are phytoestrogens or plant estrogens, which can interfere with estrogen metabolism in animals and humans. Lignans may help prevent development of certain fat and hormone sensitive types of cancer. Additionally, lignans have antibacterial, antifungal and antiviral activity. Such effects can aid the body's immune response by helping the immune system function at optimal capacity.

Studies of diet and disease risk suggest that lignans and other phytoestrogens may have anti-cancer properties. Individuals with high intakes of phytoestrogens—such as a high-fiber diet rich in lignans from vegetables and grains—have lower incidence and mortality rates of breast, endometrial and prostate cancer. Long-term studies of the effects of flaxseed in women with breast cancer are underway. (See page 19 for more information.)

Flaxseeds are among of the richest plant sources of lignans, containing from 75 to 800 times more lignans than other lignan sources. The lignan component of flaxseed makes it an even more beneficial form of nutritional supplementation than other omega-3 sources.

However, note that while flaxseed contains lignans, flaxseed oil normally does not. Some manufacturers add lignans to flaxseed oil for their health benefits. Check product packaging to determine whether flaxseed oil contains lignans.

Flaxseed and Fiber

In addition to its EFA and lignan content, flaxseed is a good source of fiber. Fiber is an important component of any diet. The 2010 Dietary Guidelines for Americans released by the United States Department of Agriculture (USDA) recommends that adults consume 14 grams of fiber for every 1,000 calories consumed. If following the typically recommended 2,000 calorie diet, most people should consume about 28 grams of fiber daily.

Several studies confirm that the soluble fiber in flaxseed can function as a cholesterol-lowering agent similar to other foods that contain soluble fiber. Because it contains omega-3 fatty acids and soluble fiber together, flaxseed presents two ingredients that favor healthy blood lipid patterns. The nutrient composition of flaxseed is given below. Keep in mind that while whole flaxseeds or ground flaxseeds (or flaxseed meal, powder or flour) are all sources of fiber, flaxseed oil does not contain fiber.

Nutrient Profile of Flaxseed per 3 oz (100 g)

Food Energy	450 calories
Fat	41 grams
Total Dietary Fiber	28 grams
Protein	20 grams

Source: *American Oil Chemists' Society*

Flaxseed contains healthy amounts of both *soluble* and *insoluble* fiber, which explains its ability to act as a laxative and relieve constipation. Soluble fiber attracts water during digestion, turning into a gel that slows digestion. Soluble fiber may help regulate blood sugar and cholesterol levels. Insoluble fiber is indigestible and passes through the digestive system in its original form. It helps food move through the stomach more quickly and adds bulk to the stool, which can help improve elimination.

In a 1997 study published in *Gastroenterology*, 55 patients with chronic constipation caused by irritable bowel syndrome consumed either 45 grams of whole flaxseed or psyllium (another plant commonly used as a laxative) per day for three months. The patients who took flaxseed reported more improvements in constipation, bloating and abdominal pain than those who took psyllium. The common dosage for using flaxseed to treat constipation is to mix two to three tablespoons of ground flaxseed with 10 times as much water. Mixing the flaxseed with sufficient water is essential; high doses of flaxseed taken without adequate water can cause bowel obstruction.

Health Benefits of Flaxseed

A balance in EFAs is necessary for many body functions. In particular, omega-3 fatty acids, such as the alpha-linolenic acid found in flaxseed, are essential for human development and important in achieving good health throughout life. The tissues of the body require the omega-3 and omega-6 fatty acids for proper functioning. Whole and ground flaxseeds also contain lignans and fiber, which show positive effects on cancer and constipation. Supplementing the diet with flaxseed oil or flaxseed can help to prevent and manage a variety of health conditions, including:

- Heart disease
- High cholesterol
- High blood pressure
- Stroke
- Cancer
- Psoriasis
- Multiple sclerosis
- Rheumatoid arthritis
- Attention deficit hyperactivity disorder

Heart Disease

Heart disease is the leading cause of death in the United States. According to the Centers for Disease Control (CDC), in 2006, heart disease accounted for a total of over six million deaths in the United States—more than one in four deaths. Although the annual rate of death from heart disease has been declining since the late 1960s, it remains the leading cause of death in the United States and a major cause in other western countries.

The good news is that people can reduce their risk of developing and dying from heart disease, as well as lower the likelihood of having a premature heart attack. While genetics influence the likelihood of developing heart disease, modifying one's lifestyle can do much to change the effects of one's genes. The most important strategy for an individual who wishes to avoid heart disease is to adopt prevention habits. Some of the most crucial prevention tactics are:

- Avoid smoking.
- Maintain a desirable blood cholesterol level (less than 200 mg/dL).
- Keep blood pressure in the normal range (120/80 or lower).
- Regularly engage in aerobic exercise.

In addition to adopting such healthy lifestyle habits, adding certain nutrients to the diet may also be helpful in reducing the risk of heart disease. Alpha-linolenic acid, the omega-3 fatty acid in flaxseed and flaxseed oil, is one dietary supplement that can lower the risk of heart disease. In a 10-year study conducted by the Department of Nutrition at the Harvard School of Public Health, researchers followed the dietary habits of women without previously diagnosed heart disease. Women with higher intakes of alpha-linolenic acid had a much lower risk of a fatal cardiac event, such as a heart attack or stroke. Consumption of alpha-linolenic acid also correlated with a slight reduction in the risk of a non-fatal cardiac event.

The alpha-linolenic acid in flaxseed may benefit heart health by fighting *atherosclerosis*, fatty deposits in artery walls that cause the artery walls to thicken. Atherosclerosis can increase the risk of heart disease by inhibiting blood flow. Omega-3 fatty acids in flaxseed may help break up the plaque that can build up in artery walls. The less plaque, the lower the risk of developing cardiovascular disease. A study published in 2009 in the *Journal of Cardiovascular Pharmacology* reported that flaxseed reduced development of atherosclerosis in rabbits by 46 percent.

High Cholesterol

Approximately one in six adults in the United States has elevated blood cholesterol levels. High blood cholesterol happens when the body cannot process all the cholesterol an individual consumes and cholesterol begins to build up in the blood. High cholesterol is associated with atherosclerosis and *arteriosclerosis*, a similar condition. In arteriosclerosis, arteries harden due to cholesterol buildup. Both conditions result in decreased blood flow to the tissues and organs and endanger the health of the heart and brain. According to the CDC, people with high cholesterol have twice the risk for heart disease as individuals with normal cholesterol.

In order to manage cholesterol levels, people often adopt a diet low in saturated fats. Diets high in fat, particularly saturated fat, are linked with high blood cholesterol levels. While adopting a diet low in saturated fats reduces the risk for heart disease, adding alpha-linolenic acid (abundant in flaxseed oil) to the diet further reduces the risk. Replacing dietary saturated fats with polyunsaturated fats, including omega-3 fatty acids, may be more beneficial than reducing saturated fats alone.

Flaxseed may help lower total cholesterol and LDL cholesterol ("bad" cholesterol) and increase HDL cholesterol ("good" cholesterol). Alpha-linolenic acid, the essential fatty acid in flaxseed and flaxseed oil, converts into EPA and DHA. Studies suggest that both EPA and DHA can help reduce blood triglycerides, increase HDL cholesterol, reduce blood pressure, reduce platelet activity and reduce neutrophil (a type of white blood cell) activity—actions that help lower the risk of coronary heart disease.

Studies support the theory that the alpha-linolenic acid found in flaxseed is beneficial to cholesterol levels. A study published in 1998 in *Nutrition Research* looked at the effect of flaxseed supplementation in postmenopausal women with high cholesterol levels. The women in the study took 38 grams of flaxseed in either bread or muffins every day for two six-week periods. The women experienced reduced total cholesterol and LDL-cholesterol levels.

A 2005 study at the Grigore T. Popa University of Medicine and Pharmacy in Romania found that flaxseed in the diet correlated with reductions in cholesterol levels in patients. The study, published in *Revista Medico-Chirurgicala a Societatii Medici si Naturalisti din Iasi* (*Journal of the Medical-Surgical Society of Physicians and Naturalists of Iasi*), divided 40 patients with high cholesterol into groups. For 60 days, the control group adopted a cholesterol-lowering diet and the test group adopted the same diet plus 20 grams of ground flaxseeds per day. After 60 days, the group that consumed flaxseed every day experienced greater reductions in total cholesterol, LDL-cholesterol and triglyceride levels than the group that did not consume flaxseed. Their ratio of total cholesterol to HDL-cholesterol also improved.

High Blood Pressure

High blood pressure affects millions of Americans. According to the American Heart Association (AHA), approximately one in three adults has high blood pressure. Healthcare practitioners are not entirely sure what causes high blood pressure—about 95 percent of the time, healthcare practitioners cannot identify a cause. However, certain risk factors increase one's chances of developing the condition. In the United States, African Americans are twice as likely as whites to develop high blood pressure. It tends to run in families and affects more men than women. Age is also a factor—people over age 35 are more likely to develop high blood pressure. Being pregnant, obese or overweight, sedentary, eating salty or fatty foods and smoking also increase the risk of developing high blood pressure.

Several of the body's systems are involved in high blood pressure, including the endocrine, cardiovascular and nervous systems. In the early 1980s, several studies suggested that the omega-3 fatty acids found in fish oils lowered blood pressure by small but statistically significant amounts. In one study, healthy males consumed fish oils or fatty fish and experienced a reduction in blood pressure. Alpha-linolenic acid, like that found in flaxseed oil, has also been suggested as a likely factor in lowering blood pressure.

In a 1990 study published in the *Journal of Human Hypertension*, 40 men with high blood pressure added either olive oil, sunflower seed oil or flaxseed oil to their diets. The researchers found that the men who took flaxseed oil experienced lowered blood pressure. A subsequent study, published in 2010 in the *Journal of the American College of Nutrition*, found that individuals who consumed a diet rich in alpha-linolenic acid from flaxseed oil experienced a significant reduction in blood pressure.

Stroke

A stroke is sometimes called a "brain attack." Strokes happen when a blood clot blocks an artery or blood vessel, interrupting blood and oxygen flow to the brain. Without oxygen, brains cells begin to die and brain damage occurs. According to the AHA, strokes are the third leading cause of death in the United States, after heart disease and cancer. Approximately 700,000 people suffer a stroke each year. Certain risks factors can increase the risk of stroke, including diabetes and a family history of stroke. Men, individuals over 55, and those who are overweight or obese or smoke are also at a higher risk. High blood pressure and high cholesterol are also considered risk factors. As mentioned, flaxseed and flaxseed oil may help decrease blood pressure and cholesterol levels, thus decreasing the risk of stroke.

An analysis published in *Stroke*, a journal published by the AHA, studied 96 men who had previously suffered strokes. The researchers found that a higher alpha-linolenic content in the men's blood cholesterol measurements was associated with a 30 percent decrease in their risk of stroke.

Rheumatoid Arthritis

About 50 million people in the United States suffer from the debilitating effects of rheumatoid arthritis, according to the CDC. The U.S. Department of Health and Human Services estimates that about one percent of the population worldwide is afflicted with the disease. Rheumatoid arthritis causes fatigue, joint pain, stiffness and muscle aches. For many people, such symptoms are debilitating and interfere with daily activities.

An EFA deficiency can cause arthritis-like symptoms, including stiff and painful joints. Supplementing the diet with EFAs can help restore the body's EFA balance, potentially helping manage rheumatoid arthritis pain. The anti-inflammatory properties of alpha-linolenic acid may be the root of its arthritis benefits.

Researchers have validated the idea that EFAs may be effective in helping relieve rheumatoid arthritis pain. Scientists at the University of Pennsylvania conducted research on the effects of alpha-linolenic acid on arthritis sufferers. Their research, published in the *Annals of Internal Medicine* in 1993, found that six out of seven patients receiving doses of alpha-linolenic acid experienced reduced inflammation of the synovial fluid in the joints. A study published in 2004 in *American Family Physician* found that individuals with rheumatoid arthritis who consumed three grams of flaxseed per day experienced reduced morning stiffness and fewer tender joints.

Multiple Sclerosis

Multiple sclerosis (MS) is a disease of the central nervous system that destroys the myelin sheaths that cover each nerve, creating inflammation. According to the National Multiple Sclerosis Society, MS affects approximately 400,000 Americans. Symptoms include blurred vision, dizziness, numbness, weakness, tremors, slurred speech and staggering. Stress and poor nutrition may contribute to the progression of the disease. Multiple sclerosis usually occurs in individuals between the ages of 25 and 40. It often goes into remission for periods of time, then reappears. The underlying cause of the disease is unknown. Researchers are still searching for a cure.

In the 1950's, Roy Swank was the first person to propose a link between fat, particularly saturated fatty acids, and MS. Physician and researcher Hugh Sinclair amplified Swank's hypothesis in 1956 in a letter to the editor of *Lancet*, the world's leading general medical journal. Sinclair warned about the "development of relative fatty acid deficiency," meaning the diminishing proportion of EFAs in the diet owing to the increased consumption of animal fats and the removal of vegetable oils in food processing. He contended that the development of "a deficiency of normal phospholipids (or presence of abnormal phospholipids) in the nervous system, causing defective structure including demyelination," was associated with a fatty acid deficiency.

Researchers are currently pursuing research inspired by the work of Swank and Sinclair, investigating the possibility that MS is at least partially caused by prostaglandin deficiency. Prostaglandins, as mentioned earlier, are created from EFAs. Because some MS patients have reduced levels of alpha-linolenic acid, flaxseed or flaxseed oil supplements may be beneficial.

Psoriasis

Psoriasis is a skin disease characterized by patches of dry, scaly skin. The dry patches occur most commonly on the knees, elbow and scalp, but can appear anywhere on the body. Symptoms often flare up and then go into remission, but the condition is incurable. An individual with psoriasis may also suffer from arthritis. Psoriasis affects approximately 7.5 million Americans, or 2.2 percent of the population, according to the National Psoriasis Foundation.

An EFA deficiency in humans can result in skin rashes that resemble eczema and psoriasis. Flaxseed oil is among the natural therapeutic agents for psoriasis because of its rich EFA content. Some psoriasis sufferers also see improvements by eliminating the harmful dietary fats found in such sources as fried foods, margarine and hydrogenated oils because such fats interfere with EFA metabolism.

A 1986 study published in *Archives of Dermatology* found that the dietary supplementation of psoriasis patients with omega-3 oil for eight weeks was accompanied by mild to moderate improvement in psoriatic lesions in eight out of 13 patients. Two patients reported significant alleviation of their symptoms.

In 2011, a study published in *Clinical, Cosmetic and Investigational Dermatology* studied the effect of omega-3 supplementation on individuals with psoriasis. Researchers found that individuals who took an omega-3 supplement had better results than the control group that did not take omega-3 supplements.

Studies also suggest that adding omega-3 fatty acids to topical treatments can also be beneficial. Try adding flaxseed oil to a cream or a lotion and applying to affected skin, or apply flaxseed oil straight onto the skin. Combining internal and external use of flaxseed oil may be particularly helpful.

Cancer

Scientists at the American National Cancer Institute singled out flaxseed as one of six foods that deserved special study due to potential cancer-fighting ability. Certain types of fats have been linked with the development of malignancies (cancer cells that spread). Evidence suggests that obtaining a consistent supply of omega-3 oils may help prevent certain fat-sensitive types of cancer. One interesting property of omega-3 fatty acids is their ability to neutralize the undesirable effects of detrimental fatty acids found in certain vegetables and meats.

Because some cancers need certain hormones to grow, cancer researchers have largely focused on the lignan component of flaxseed in cancer prevention. Lignans may prevent estrogen from affecting breast cancer cells. Although the exact mechanism is unclear, researchers have found that flaxseed has the potential to reduce tumor growth in patients with breast cancer. A 1994 study published in *Breast Cancer Journal* studied flaxseed's potential to reduce tumor growth. Researchers studied 121 patients with breast cancer over a 31-month follow-up period. The researchers found that lower levels of alpha-linolenic acid correlated with larger tumor sizes and the development of metastasis, the process by which cancer spreads.

In a more recent study, published in 2005 in *Clinical Cancer Research*, researchers studied 32 postmenopausal women with newly diagnosed breast cancer. The researchers divided the women into either a treatment or placebo group. The treatment group received a muffin containing 25 grams of flaxseed per day, while the control group received muffins with no flaxseed. The researchers found that the women who ate the flaxseed muffins had higher levels of lignans (according to urinary analysis). Higher lignan levels correlated with reduced tumor growth in the women.

One significant study also suggests that flaxseed may be beneficial in reducing the risk of prostate cancer, or in reducing cancer growth in patients with prostate cancer. The 2008 study, funded by the National Institute of Health and published in *Clinical Trials*, combined flaxseed supplementation (30 grams per day) and dietary fat restriction. The study followed 161 patients who were scheduled for surgical removal of the prostate gland. The researchers concluded that flaxseed may have had a protective effect against prostate cancer and that the greatest benefit may come from combining intake of flaxseed with a low fat diet.

Attention Deficit Hyperactivity Disorder

According to the CDC, approximately 5.4 million children between the ages of four and 17 had attention deficit hyperactivity disorder (ADHD) in 2007. ADHD is a developmental disorder that most commonly affects children, although it affects teens and adults as well. According to the National Institute of Mental Health, ADHD symptoms include, "difficulty staying focused and paying attention, difficulty controlling behavior, and hyperactivity." Preliminary experimental and clinical evidence suggests that a deficiency or imbalance in EFAs can contribute to ADHD.

A pilot study published in 2006 in *Prostaglandins, Leukotrienes and Essential Fatty Acids* tested the effect of flaxseed oil supplementation on children with ADHD. Clinicians reported that children who took flaxseed oil supplements experienced reduced ADHD symptoms, according to total hyperactivity scores on an ADHD rating scale. Flaxseed oil may be a promising dietary supplement in reducing symptoms of ADHD, although more studies are needed to confirm results.

Additional Roles of Flaxseed and Flaxseed Oil

So far, we've discussed some impressive conclusions about the health benefits of flaxseed oil. But that's just the tip of the iceberg. Because flaxseed research is in its infancy, additional uses will likely be uncovered in the future. Below is a summary of some uses for which flaxseed is beginning to be recognized as useful therapy.

Allergies: Allergies are the immune system's abnormal response to substances that are usually harmless. A substance that causes an allergic response is called an allergen. When an allergen comes in contact with the skin or eyes or is inhaled, the body responds by releasing hormones that cause inflammation. The body's inflammatory response causes the symptoms associated with allergies, including itchiness, runny nose, congestion or hives. As an omega-3 fatty acid, alpha-linolenic acid works to reduce the body's inflammatory response and may help manage allergy symptoms.

Constipation: Constipation is generally defined as having fewer than three bowel movements per week. According to the National Digestive Diseases Information Clearinghouse, constipation is one of the most common gastrointestinal complaints in the United States. One of the most common causes of constipation is insufficient fiber in the diet. As a good source of dietary fiber, flaxseed may help decrease symptoms of constipation. A 1997 study published in *Gastroenterology* found that flaxseed can help manage symptoms of constipation in individuals suffering from irritable bowel syndrome.

Consuming flaxseed daily can increase the frequency of bowel movements. As a laxative, the traditional dose is two to three tablespoons of ground flaxseed mixed in 10 times the amount of water. Grinding the flaxseed improves absorption, as whole flaxseed may pass through the digestive tract undigested, producing no benefit.

Cyclic mastalgia (breast pain): Many women experience cyclic mastalgia (breast pain and tenderness in connection with fluctuating hormones related to the monthly menstrual cycle). According to a study published in *Breast Cancer Research Treatment* in 2000, flaxseed lignans may help reduce estrogen levels, which in turn may reduce breast pain, swelling and lumps, all symptoms of cyclic mastalgia. Studies generally use flaxseed muffins containing 25 to 50 grams of flaxseed to treat breast pain.

Diabetes: The omega-3 oils in flaxseed have been shown to lower insulin requirements in some individuals. Any diabetic patient wishing to take flaxseed should monitor blood glucose levels carefully, just as with any other dietary supplement. Flaxseed and flaxseed oil can also aid in circulation, which is an important factor in diabetes. Studies generally use flaxseed muffins containing 25 to 50 grams of flaxseed in people with diabetes.

Dry eye syndrome (keratoconjunctivitis sicca): Dry eye syndrome is a disease caused by either decreased tear production or increased tear film evaporation. In either case, individuals suffering from dry eye syndrome experience dryness, burning and a feeling of having sand or grit in the eye that typically worsens as the day goes on. Dry eye syndrome can cause damage to the eye that results in sensitivity to light and further discomfort. Approximately four million Americans suffer from dry eye syndrome. According to a study published in 2007 in *Arquivos Brasileiros de Oftalmologia* (*Brazilian Archives of Ophthalmology*), one to two grams of flaxseed oil per day taken orally may help alleviate inflammation associated with dry eye syndrome.

HIV/AIDS: Lignans found in flaxseed show promise in helping manage HIV/AIDS. AIDS, or acquired immunodeficiency syndrome, is an autoimmune disease caused by the human immunodeficiency virus (HIV). The virus gradually destroys the function of the immune system by infecting healthy immune system cells and causing them to mutate. Once the virus has caused one cell to mutate, it can spread and cause other cells to mutate. In a study published in *AIDS Research and Human Retroviruses*, researchers found that lignans appeared to inhibit replication of HIV.

One common symptom of HIV is weight loss and inability to gain weight. In one study, published in 1996 in the *Journal of the American Dietetic Association*, HIV patients took a fortified formula containing alpha-linolenic acid, arginine and yeast RNA for four months. While taking the formula, the patients were able to gain weight. Because the formula contained three substances, the effects are not necessarily attributable entirely to flaxseed, but the results are promising. Researchers are still investigating other potential health benefits of lignans, but lignans show promise in cancer treatment and prevention, HIV/AIDS treatment and many other benefits.

Menopause: Menopause symptoms such as mood swings, hot flashes and weight gain affect tens of thousands of women. In addition, many women experience increases in cholesterol along with menopause. Due to its alpha-linolenic acid and lignan content, flaxseed may help manage such irritating and painful symptoms. In a study published in *Obstetrics and Gynecology* in 2002, researchers looked at the effect of incorporating flaxseed into the diet of 199 menopausal women. The researchers found that flaxseed reduced severity of hot flashes and night sweats. Additionally, the researchers reported that the women consuming flaxseed also experienced reductions in cholesterol levels.

Osteoporosis: Osteoporosis is a major health concern for 44 million Americans age 50 and over, according to the National Osteoporosis Foundation. That means that approximately 55 percent of the population over age 50 is affected by osteoporosis. Individuals with osteoporosis have low bone mass that causes bones to be weak and easy to break. Bones may become brittle as a result of too little calcium in the diet, or the bones may not adequately absorb calcium.

A 2001 study published in *Alternative Medicine Review* suggested that including omega-3s as part of the diet or in dietary supplements may slow bone loss. The researchers found that flaxseed and flaxseed oil supplements may help increase calcium absorption, bone calcium and bone density.

Continuing Research

Researchers continue to discover additional benefits of flaxseed and flaxseed oil. Recently, researchers have also found that dietary supplementation with flaxseed oil reduces the production of cytokines—agents that can suppress or boost immune system function. Some anti-inflammatory pharmaceuticals inhibit the production of cytokines, but flaxseed oil may be a natural alternative to pharmaceutical anti-inflammatory medications.

Ongoing research suggests that EFAs play an important role for normal function during growth and development of infants and in the mediation of chronic disease. Thus, infants and pregnant and lactating women may benefit from including EFAs in their diets. Researchers suggest that a diet balanced with omega-3 and omega-6 fatty acids may delay or decrease the manifestation of many diseases, including cardiovascular disease, hypertension and autoimmune, allergic and neurological disorders. With its optimal ratio of omega-6 to omega-3 fatty acids, flaxseed offers an excellent option for individuals trying to support a healthy EFA balance in the body.

Selecting a Flaxseed Source

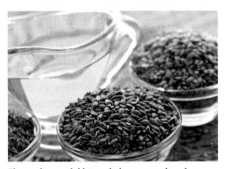

Flaxseed is available as whole or ground seeds.

Essential fatty acids are fragile and easily damaged by air, high temperatures and food processing. Unfortunately, most of the oils available today have been heavily processed by heat and filtering processes, which change the structure of fatty acids and can remove beneficial substances such as lignans. Therefore, choosing flaxseed or flaxseed oil that have not been damaged by processing is very important. In addition, keep in mind the different advantages of taking flaxseed oil versus flaxseed itself: flaxseed oil contains alpha-linolenic acid, but does not contain fiber or lignans, while whole or crushed flaxseed contain alpha-linolenic acid, dietary fiber and lignans.

Choosing a Good Flaxseed Oil

Not all flaxseed oils are created equal. Quality and purity can vary tremendously as a result of differences in how the oil is expressed, or extracted, from the seed. Most flaxseed oils are produced by mechanically pressing the seeds through an expeller. Pressing can generate a tremendous amount of pressure and heat. The higher the heat, the higher the yield of oil. Temperatures generally reach 200 degrees Fahrenheit. Flaxseed oil processed in such a manner can still be referred to as cold-pressed because no external source of heat is added.

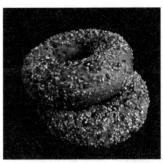

Flaxseed pumps up the nutrition of breads, pastas, oatmeal and more!

However, as mentioned, flaxseed oil is extremely susceptible to damage by heat, light and oxygen. Hence, although high temperatures will provide a greater quantity of oil, they produce lower quality oil. Many manufacturers sacrifice quality for quantity.

The preferred method of safely extracting flaxseed oil uses a special expeller that keeps temperatures below six degrees Fahrenheit. Keeping temperatures low helps protect the delicate oil from the damaging effects of heat.

One of the best ways to measure the quality of flaxseed oil is by taste. The degree of bitterness is a close approximation of the level of lipid peroxides, which are toxic molecules. Avoid flaxseed oil that tastes bitter or rancid.

A few things to look for when purchasing flaxseed oil:

- Find a flaxseed oil derived from 100 percent third-party certified organic flaxseed. Oil expressed from non-organic flaxseed may contain pesticides and herbicides.
- Make sure the oil is as fresh as possible and not past the expiration date.
- Check the label to be sure it clearly indicates that the oil is expeller-pressed, not extracted using heat or a solvent method (which uses hexane, a poisonous chemical).
- Flaxseed oil should be refrigerated in an opaque bottle, which protects the oil from the heat, light and oxygen.
- For the greatest benefit, look for a flaxseed oil high in lignans. Most flaxseed oils do not contain lignans, but some manufacturers process the oil and include particles of flaxseeds to capture the lignan content. The bottle will indicate whether the manufacturer included lignans.

Tips for Storing and Using Whole or Ground Flaxseed

Ground flaxseed, milled flaxseed and flaxseed meal are all the same thing. Nutritionists recommend using ground forms instead of whole flaxseed because they are easier for the body to digest. You can buy ground flaxseed, or grind your own using a coffee grinder. Some blenders also have a special dry blade that can be used to grind flaxseed. Whole flaxseeds can be stored in a dark, cool and dry place for up to one year. Ground flaxseeds can be stored in a refrigerator for up to three months, or in a freezer for six months.

Whole or ground flaxseeds can be mixed with water or juice and taken as a drink, or mixed and baked into other foods. Flaxseed can be baked into muffins or sprinkled on top of cereal or fruit. Following are some tips for how to add more flaxseed to your diet.

- **Add flaxseed to your daily routine.** An easy way to incorporate flaxseed into your diet is to add one to two tablespoons of ground flaxseed or flaxseed oil to foods you normally eat. You can add flaxseed to oatmeal, smoothies, soup, yogurt and more!
- **Mix it into main dishes.** Ground flaxseed mixes well with dishes that are moist and darker in color. A few tablespoons of ground flaxseed can add fiber and nutrition to chili, casseroles, stew, meatloaf and more.
- **Bake with it.** Flaxseed is delicious in baked goods such as quick breads, muffins, waffles and cookies.

Precautions with Whole and Ground Flaxseed

Consuming flaxseed in whole or ground form at the same time as other oral medications may decrease absorption of oral medications, vitamins or minerals. Take all oral medications one hour before or two hours after taking flaxseed to prevent decreased absorption. Flaxseed oil does not decrease or prevent absorption of oral medications.

Dosing

As a general rule, consult a healthcare practitioner before taking any dietary supplement, including flaxseed or flaxseed oil. The following are dosing suggestions for different forms of flaxseed and flaxseed oil.

Flaxseed oil: Most nutritionists and health care providers recommend one tablespoon of flaxseed oil for every 100 pounds of body weight, to be used daily. For a child, the recommended dose is one teaspoon of flaxseed oil for every 33 pounds of body weight.

Flaxseed oil capsules: The advantage of flaxseed oil capsules is their convenience—they are very convenient for traveling and for keeping in places where refrigeration is not possible. However, it takes about 14 capsules to equal one tablespoon of liquid flaxseed oil since each a tablespoon is equivalent to 14 grams and capsules typically contain one gram of flaxseed oil.

Flaxseed: A standard dose is one to two tablespoons of ground flaxseed per day.

Promote Whole Body Health

Because of its high omega-3 fatty acid content in the form of alpha-linolenic acid, flaxseed and flaxseed oil have a wide array of health benefits. The omega-3 fatty acids in flaxseed and flaxseed oil are important because they are essential nutrients often lacking in the standard American diet. The omega-3s in flaxseed are particularly attractive for vegans and vegetarians, who often do not get enough omega-3 fatty acids, as such nutrients typically come from fish sources.

In addition to being an agent in the prevention of heart disease, flaxseed and flaxseed oil can help improve skin problems and auto-immune disorders. Perhaps its greatest value lies in its ability to fight cancer due to its abundance of lignans. And flaxseed is a well-known source of healthy dietary fiber, which aids in relieving constipation among other benefits. Flaxseed and flaxseed oil supplementation can help the body function at an optimum performance level.

References

Arjmandi B.H., D.A. Khan, et al. "Whole flaxseed consumption lowers serum LDL-cholesterol and lipoprotein(a) concentrations in postmenopausal women." *Nutrition Research* 18 no. 7 (1998): 1203–14.

Balbás G.M., M.S. Regaña, et al. "Study on the use of omega-3 fatty acids as a therapeutic supplement in treatment of psoriasis." *Clinical, Cosmetic and Investigational Dermatology* 4 (2011): 73–7.

Barlean's Organic Oils, LLC. "Flaxseed oil and fish oil: values of the omega-3 family." Accessed June 17, 2011. http://www.barleans.com/literature/flax/21-nothing-fishy.html.

Bougnoux, P., S. Koscielny, et al. "Alpha-Linolenic acid content of adipose breast tissue: a host determinant of the risk of early metastasis in breast cancer." *Breast Cancer Journal* 70, no. 2 (1994): 330–4.

Chan, J.K., B.E. McDonale, et al. "Effect of dietary alpha-linolenic acid and its ratio to linolenic acid on platelet and plasma fatty acids and thrombogenesis." *Lipids* 28 (1993): 811–7.

Clark, W. F., A. Parbtani, et al. "Flaxseed: a potential treatment for lupus nephritis." *Kidney International* 48, no. 2 (1995): 475–80.

Covington M.B. "Omega-3 fatty acids." *American Family Physician* 70, no. 1 (July 2004): 133–40.

Ddyken, M.L., P.A. Wolf, et al. "Risk Factors in Stroke: a statement for physicians by the subcommittee on risk factors and stroke of the stroke council." *Stroke* 15 (1984): 1105–11.

Demark-Wahnefried, W., S.L. George, et al. "Overcoming challenges in designing and implementing a phase II randomized controlled trial using a presurgical model to test a dietary intervention in prostate cancer." *Clinical Trials* 5, no. 3 (2008): 262–72.

Flax Council of Canada. "Flax Nutrition Profile." Accessed on July 2, 2011. http://www.flaxcouncil.ca/english/index.jsp?p=g3&mp=nutrition.

Goss P.E., T. Li, et al. "Effects of dietary flaxseed in women with cyclical mastalgia." *Breast Cancer Research Treatment* 64 (2000): 49.

Guyenet, S. "Omega-6 Linoleic Acid Suppresses Thyroid Signaling." *Whole Health Source: Ancestral Nutritional and Health* (blog), Dec. 19, 2008, http://wholehealthsource.blogspot.com/2008/12/omega-6-linoleic-acid-suppresses.html.

Hu, F. B., M.J. Stampfer, et al. "Dietary intake of alpha-linolenic acid and risk of fatal ischemic heart disease among women." *American Journal of Clinical Nutrition* 69, no. 5 (1999): 890-897.

Joshi, K., S. Lad, et al. "Supplementation with flaxseed oil and vitamin C improves the outcome of Attention Deficit Hyperactivity Disorder (ADHD)." *Prostaglandins, Leukotrienes and Essential Fatty Acids* 74, no. 1 (2006): 17-21.

Kettler D.B. "Can manipulation of the ratios of essential fatty acids slow the rapid rate of postmenopausal bone loss?" *Alternative Medicine Review* 6, no. 1 (2001): 61-77.

Lai P.K., J. Donovan, et al. "Modification of human immunodeficiency viral replication by pine cone extracts." *AIDS Research and Human Retroviruses* 6, no. 2 (Feb. 1990): 205-17.

Lemay A, S. Dodin, et al. "Flaxseed dietary supplement versus hormone replacement therapy in hypercholesterolemic menopausal women." *Obstetrics and Gynecology* 100, no. 3 (Sept. 2002): 495-504.

Leventhal L.J., E.G. Boyce EG, et al. "Treatment of rheumatoid arthritis with gamma linolenic acid." *Annals of Internal Medicine* 119, no. 9 (Nov. 1993): 867-73.

Magee, Elaine, MPH, RD. "Benefits of Flaxseed." Accessed on June 29, 2011. http://www.webmd.com/diet/features/benefits-of-flaxseed.

Mandaşescu S., V. Mocanu, et al. "Flaxseed supplementation in hyperlipidemic patients." *Revista Medico-Chirurgicala a Societatii Medici si Naturalisti din Iasi* 109, no. 3 (Jul–Sept. 2005): 502–6.

Murphy R.A., M. Mourtzakis, et al. "Nutritional intervention with fish oil provides a benefit over standard of care for weight and skeletal muscle mass in patients with nonsmall cell lung cancer receiving chemotherapy." *Cancer* 117, no. 8 (April 15, 2011): 1775–82.

National Center for Complementary and Alternative Medicine. "Flaxseed and flaxseed oil." Last modified July 2010. http://nccam.nih.gov/health/flaxseed/ataglance.htm.

National Institute of Mental Health. "What is Attention Deficit Hyperactivity Disorder?" Last modified on January 23, 2009. http://www.nimh.nih.gov/health/publications/attention-deficit-hyperactivity-disorder-easy-to-read/index.shtml.

Natural Standard. 2011. Professional Monograph: "Flaxseed and flaxseed oil (*Linum usitatissimum*)." http://naturalstandard.com/databases/herbssupplements/flaxseed.asp.

Pinheiro, M.N., Jr., P.M. dos Santos, et al. "Oral flaxseed oil (*Linum usitatissimum*) in the treatment for dry-eye Sjogren's syndrome patients." *Arquivos Brasileiros de Oftalmologia* 70, no. 4 (2007): 649–55.

Prasad K. "Flaxseed and cardiovascular health." *Journal of Cardiovascular Pharmacology* 54, no. 5 (Nov. 2009): 369–77.

Suttmann, U., J. Ockenga, et al. "Weight gain and increased concentrations of receptor proteins for tumor necrosis factor after patients with symptomatic HIV infection received fortified nutrition support." *Journal of the American Dietetic Association* 96, no. 6 (1996): 565–9.

Tarpila, S. and A. Kivinen. "Ground flaxseed is an effective hypolipidemic bulk laxative." *Gastroenterology* 112 (1997): A836.

Thompson, L.U., J.M. Chen, et al. "Dietary flaxseed alters tumor biological markers in postmenopausal breast cancer." *Clinical Cancer Research* 11, no. 10 (2005): 3828–35.

West S.G., A.L. Krick, et al. "Effects of diets high in walnuts and flax oil on hemodynamic responses to stress and vascular endothelial function." *Journal of the American College Nutrition* 29, no. 6 (Dec. 2010): 595–603.

Ziboh, V.A., K.A. Cohen, et al. "Effects of dietary supplementation of fish oil on neutrophil and epidermal fatty acids: modulation of the clinical course of psoriatic subjects." *Archives of Dermatology* 122 (1986): 1277–81.